SMART GUIDE TO FRAGRANCE SHOPPING: by a Perfume Spritzer.

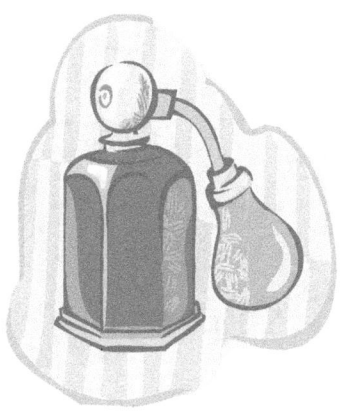

Author: Irene Sangwa

Http://www.theperfumespritzer.com

This booklet is dedicated to all my
fellow Perfume Models and sales
associates.

ACKNOWLEDGEMENTS

I would like to thank those who were helpful in getting this guide completed. First and foremost, a big thank you to all my friends; without you, there would be no guide. To Rosa, for her counsel. To my dear friend X, thank you for keeping me on track. To big Ed, thank you for helping me "run".

Coming soon: The mini tales of the Perfume Spitzer"

CONTENTS

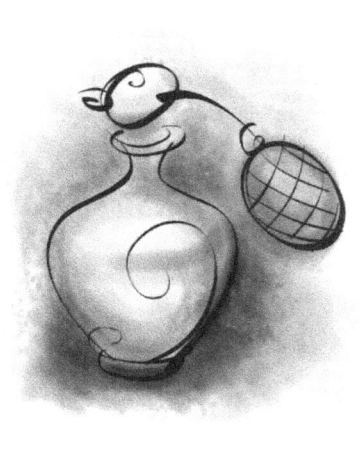

DO YOUR HOMEWORK

When in the market for a new scent, the magazines and the internet are your best source of information on the subject. Use them! If you are looking for the latest and greatest in fragrance, make sure to always pay attention to the beauty section of your favorite magazine as well.

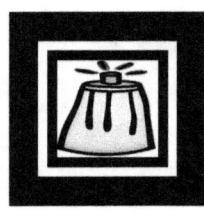
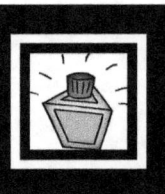
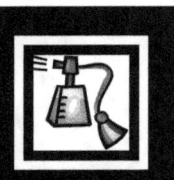
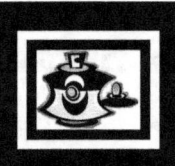
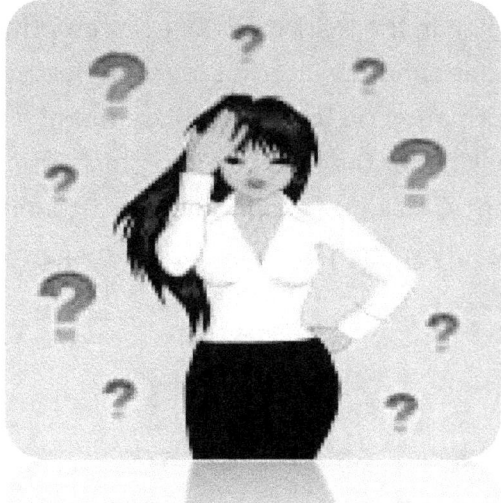

KNOW WHAT YOU LIKE!

Find out what type of scent or smell you are the most attracted to; floral, fruity, spicy, woody...

Sometimes, it is as simple as going to your local flower shop and getting yourself familiarize with the different type of flower scents. Your local spice shop is also a great place to experiment. You can also do the same thing in the comfort of your own home; use what you have around you, be it the fruits in your kitchen, the smell of a leather belt or your new purse. Ask yourself how you feel about those scents.

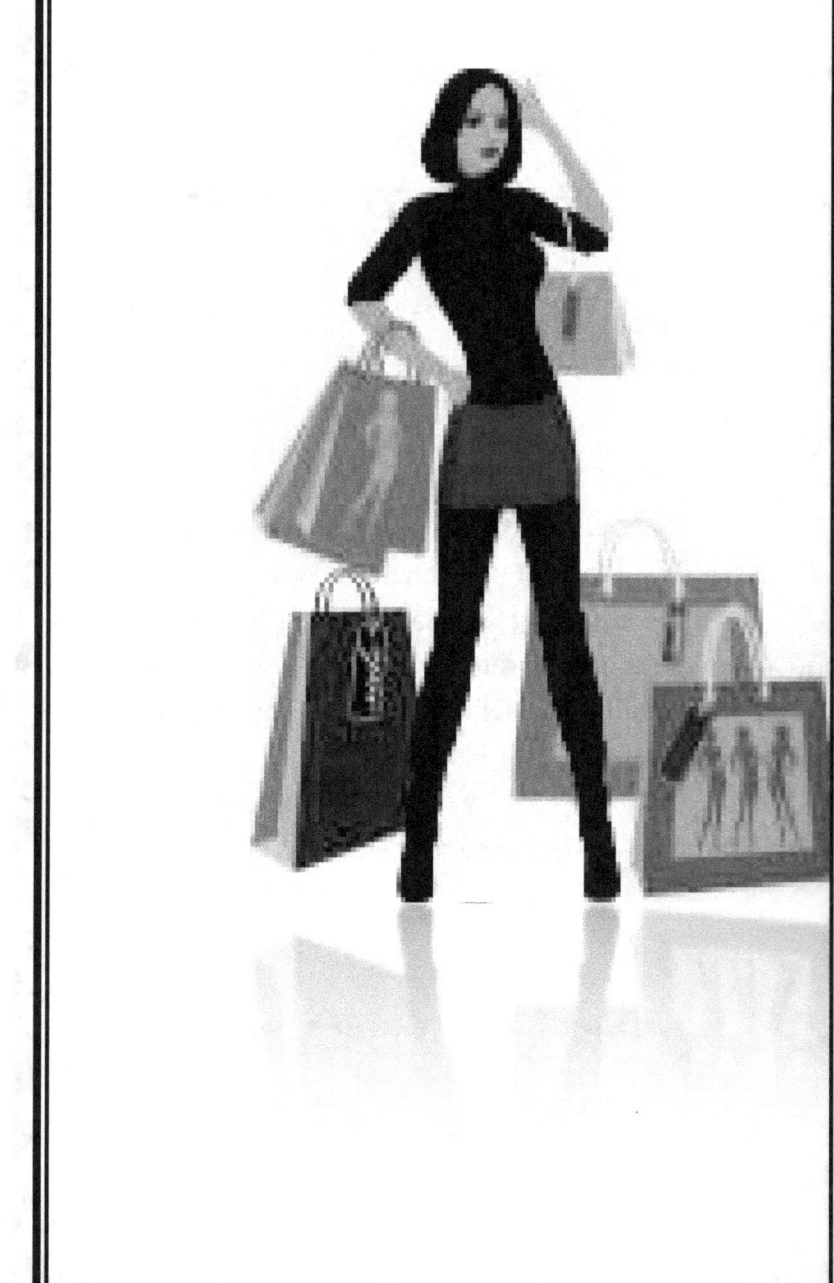

KNOW WHAT YOU DON'T WANT!

It is easy to feel a bit overwhelmed when you first walk in a fragrance department and you are faced with a multitude of choices and all the pretty bottles. Don't let it stop you; this is where your initial research comes in handy.

If you are not sure where to start, take a deep breath and ask for guidance; there is always someone around to help you with your search.

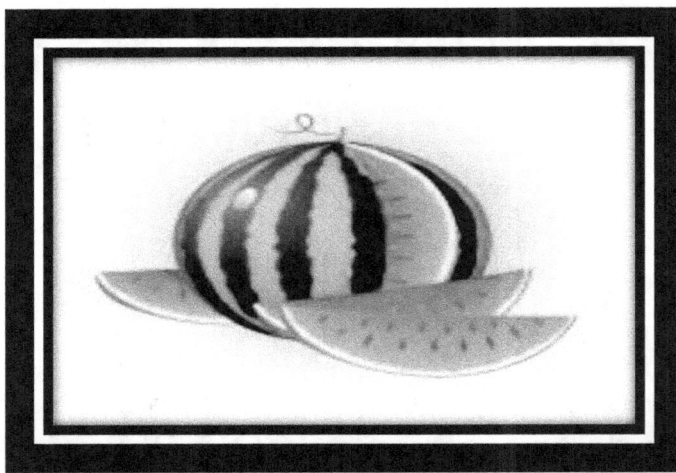

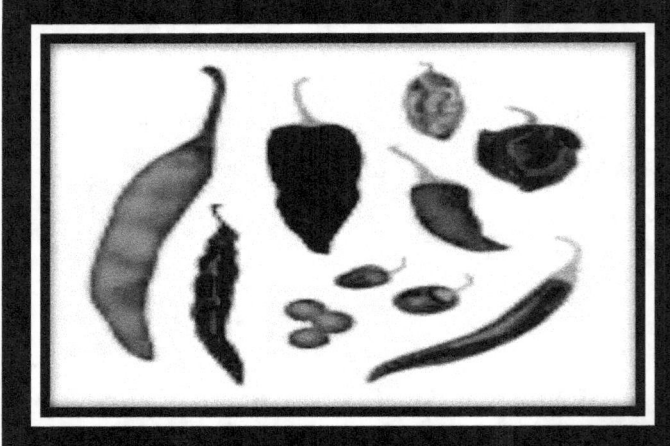

NOTES?

The shop owner, sales associate, perfume models are trained on each product, but sometimes they forget certain notes in a scent. It is in your best interest to ask specific questions.

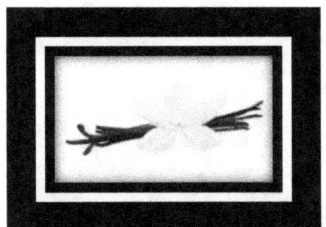

Most stores are equipped with computers and internet. If you are not sure about all the notes in a fragrance, they can also look them up for you.

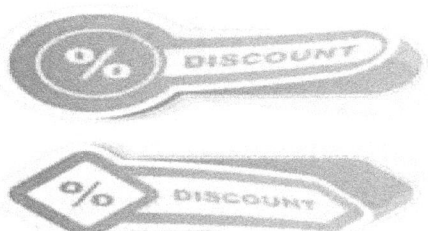

Discounts and gifts with purchase…

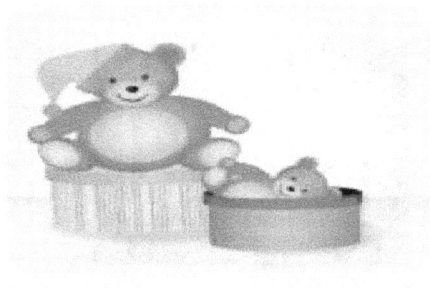

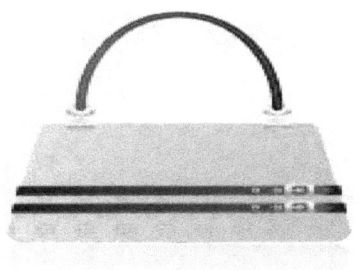

GIFT WITH PURCHASE

The gifts with purchase or GWP, as we commonly call them are a great incentive after you've made your purchase. When shopping for your fragrance, try not to focus too much on the size of the gift or the quality of the gift. Stay focus on your purchase; the goal is for you to end up with a product you will enjoy and will want to replenish when needed.

Once you've found the fragrance that matches your personality, the sales associate will make sure to give you your GWP as a reward for you business.

Sometimes, the person ringing your purchase might forget to give you a gift; kindly remind them.

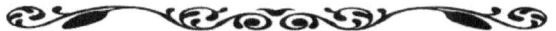

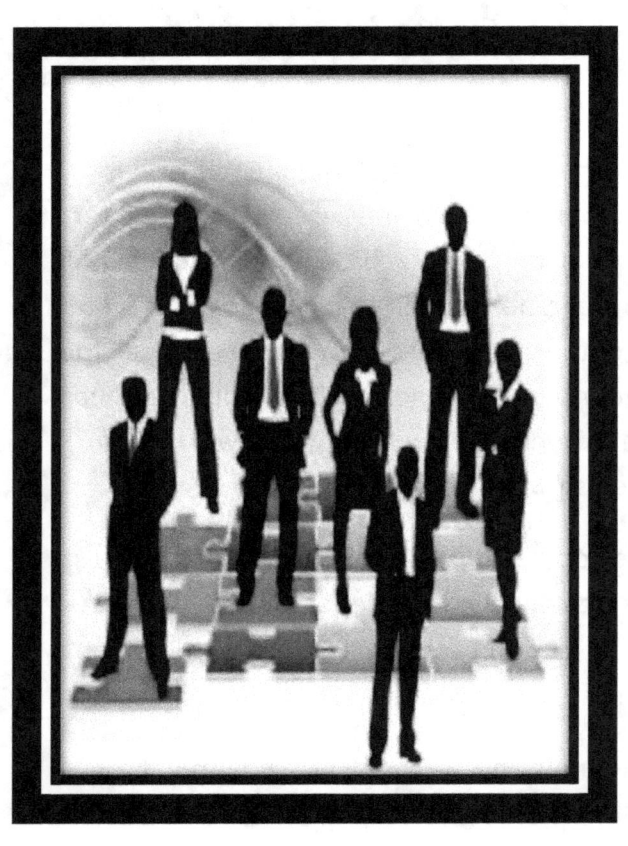

THE SALES ASSOCIATES.

Yes, at times it can be a bit intimidating to see a group of people in the fragrance area of the store; just know that they are not obstacles. These people are there for your benefit. They are highly qualified in what they do. Think of them as facilitators. They take pride in what they do and their desire is to help you.

They know what's old, what's new, and what's hot... Feel free to ask for their suggestion or opinion on a specific product you've picked; they will help. They want you to be happy and satisfied with your choice of fragrance. A happy customer always comes back!

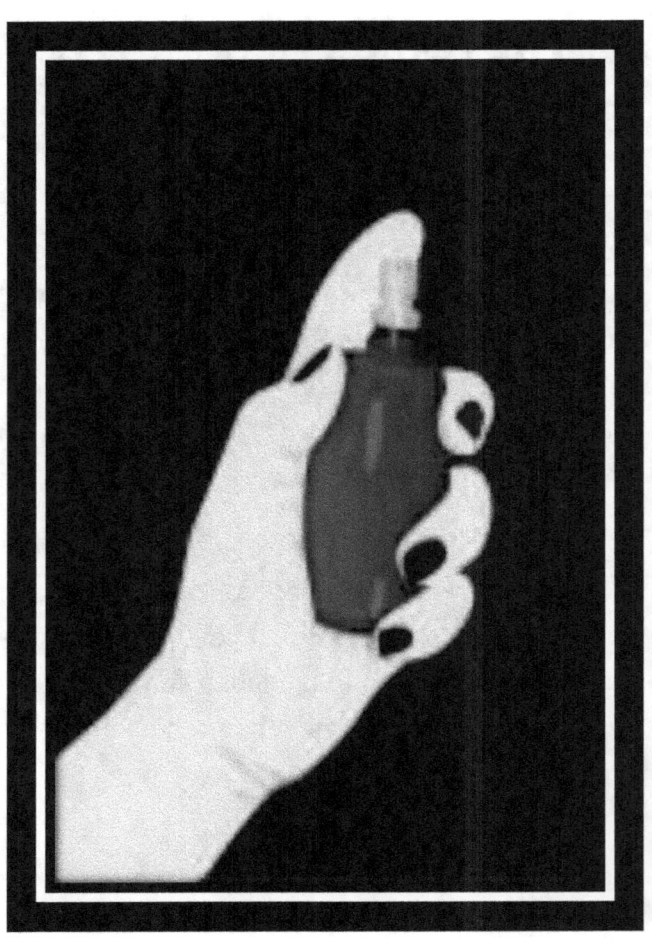

SPRAYING YOU.

Sometimes, it is in your best interest that we spray you; this is the best way for you (the client) to really see how the "dream juice" will work on your skin. Don't be defensive when you see a Perfume Model or a sales associate holding a bottle of fragrance; most of them rarely spray because of allergies.

Once you have narrowed your choices down to two or three, you should definitely try it; at least on your pinky finger, that way, if you don't like the scent on your finger, you can ask for a baby wipe and clean it off. Most stores have them on hand. You can then repeat the experiment until you have found the scent that suits you.

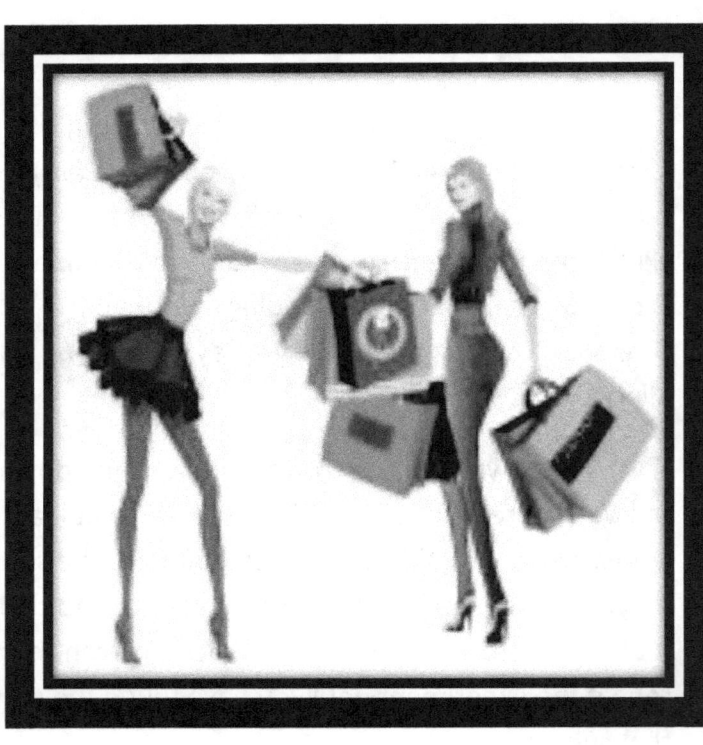

YOUR FRIENDS OPINION.

We all love our friends and value their opinion. When it comes to picking a fragrance, I recommend that you rely on your own judgment. Our skins are not made equal; therefore the scent you love on your friend or coworker might not be the perfect fit for you.

Your friends can help you create a list of fragrances that you can try or experiment with. The list is only a tool to guide you in your search; just remember that you don't have to like what your friend likes. Be your own person.

Monday

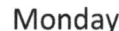

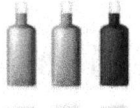

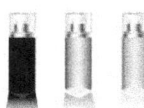

Wednesday

Friday

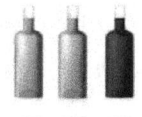

Sunday

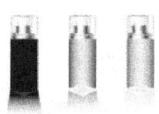

Tuesday

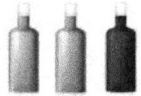

SAMPLES.

Fragrance samples are a great tool when used properly. Once you've narrowed your search down to hopefully two or three choices that you might like, ask the sales associate or the perfume spritzer if there are any samples available for you to try home.

If you decide to purchase one of your three choices, don't hesitate to ask for a sample of the other two fragrances you picked. Who knows, you might just decide later on to come back and purchase them to add to your new collection. If there aren't any samples available, once again, use your pinky finger; it helps!

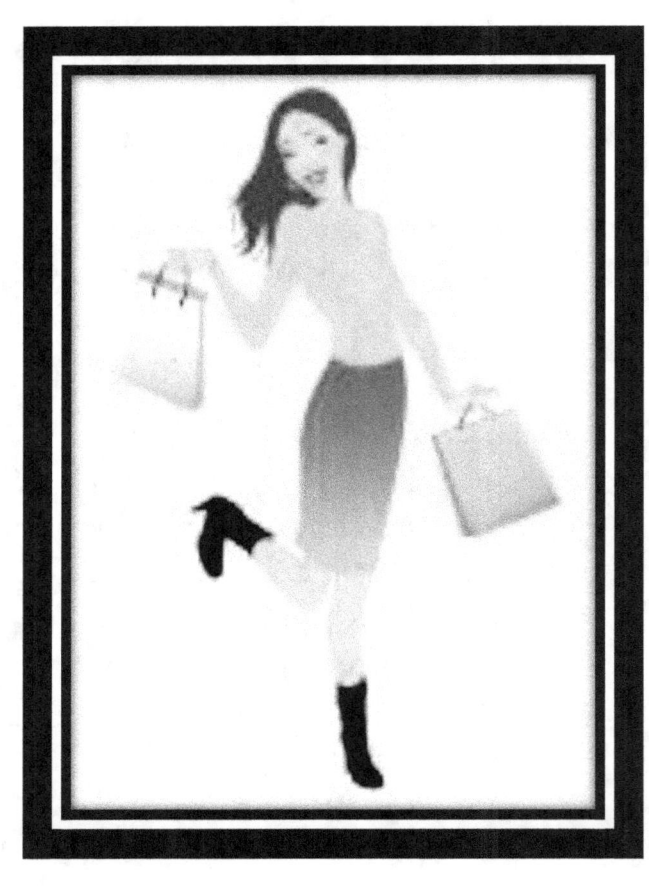

CONCLUSION

Fragrance shopping does not have to be a dreaded experience.

Just remember that you are not purchasing something as important as a car, and there is no such thing as picking the "wrong" fragrance. You can always return it, give it away, or just keep it as a souvenir.

Now go out and have fun shopping for your dream juice!

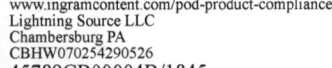